The Plant-Based Paleo Diet Guide

I0441448

Enjoy the Health Benefits of Eating the Caveman Way

RON KNESS

Contents

Disclaimer

This publication is for informational purposes only and is not intended as medical advice. Medical advice should always be obtained from a qualified medical professional for any health conditions or symptoms associated with them.

Every possible effort has been made in preparing and researching this material. We make no warranties with respect to the accuracy, applicability of its contents or any omissions.

See your healthcare professional before starting any diet or exercise program!

Introduction: What is the Paleo Diet?

Have you heard about the caveman diet? It is also known as the Paleo diet, because it mimics the foods that humans ate during the Paleolithic era. Contrary to popular belief, the Paleo Diet is not totally plant-based. Yes, humans during this prehistory did eat whatever plants, fruits and vegetables were available to them. But they ate a lot of meat as well.

As a matter of fact, they ate whatever they could whenever they had a chance. This period of time saw humans learn to make and use stone tools, and begin to form bands or groups. This was the beginning of societies as we know them today. They gathered plants, hunted and fished, and it was during this very influential age of man that art, religion and spiritual practices first developed.

These humans who lived 15,000 years ago ate only natural foods. This was pre-agriculture and pre-dairy. Obviously, there were no industries and corporations spewing unhealthy pollution into the air and water. There were no McDonald's or Starbucks

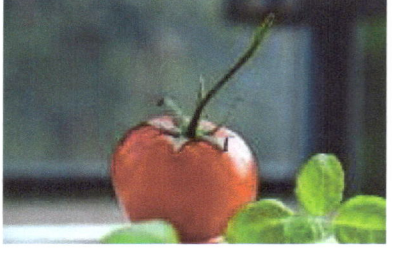

stores pumping garbage into Paleolithic man either. He enjoyed a healthy diet of fish, seeds, fruits and meat, and truly "lived off of the land".

That simple nutrition plan means that only natural foods entered the human body.

Why is that important? Well, scientists have studied the remains of human beings from the Paleolithic time period, and found something very startling.

These humans didn't suffer from diabetes, high blood pressure, cholesterol problems, obesity and heart disease.

Those dangerous and deadly conditions began to pop up when humans began eating wheat. Massive droughts in Europe and other areas around the world meant that humans had to eat what was available ... and at that time, there was plenty of wheat. Wheat was mixed with water, and this was the origin of today's bread. Experimentation led to the basis of unhealthy foods and food components we know today, such as trans fats, processed foods, processed sugars and simple carbohydrates.

This drastic shift in the human diet meant that people did not have to hunt and roam for their food anymore. But since they turned away from the fish, meats, seeds, fruit and nuts that made up the Paleolithic diet, this led to many of the diseases we know today.

Protein will be as much as 30% of your daily eating plan, with as much as 45% or 50% of your calories coming from carbohydrates delivered in the form of high fiber fruits and vegetables. As much as 25% to 45% of your calories will come from healthy fats.

For a hard definition, you can consider the Paleo diet as ...

"A nutritional approach to eating that adopts the diet of Paleolithic man. Vegetables, leafy greens, seeds, meats, fish and nuts comprise that diet."

Then Isn't A Plant-Based Paleo Diet Impossible?

Many people believe that the Paleo diet is not possible if you'd prefer to eat plant-based, but this isn't true. Of course, you won't be able to stick to the strict definition of the Paleo diet that we just shared, but the Paleo diet principles can be taken and adapted to those who do not consume animal products. This guide will show you how.

First, we will cover the main principles of Paleo food, and

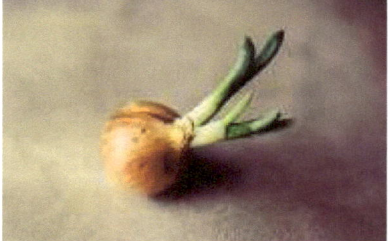

then we will learn how to adapt them to both a vegetarian and a vegan diet. Finally, we will share *why* it's we'll worth considering the plant-based or "Pegan" version of a Paleo diet.

Let's get started!

What Foods Are Allowed on the Paleo Diet?

Research shows us that approximately 73% of the American diet consists of processed foods. Guess what? Those are not allowed on the caveman diet. Just think about what was available to primitive man before the invention of pizza, cheeseburgers, chocolate cake and anything covered with gravy.

The Stone Age diet allows you to eat the following foods:

- Eggs (no more than 6 to 12 per week, aim for Omega-3 enriched eggs, if at all possible)

- Nuts and seeds (no more than 4 ounces a day if you are trying to lose weight. Raw, unsalted nuts were available to prehistoric man, so that is what you will be eating.)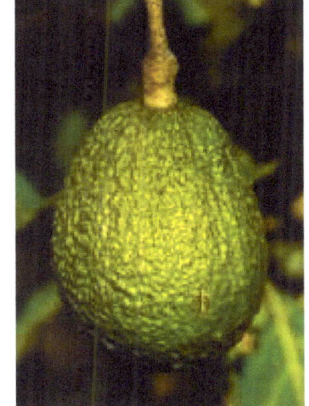

- Healthy fats, like those found in olive oil, coconut oil, avocados and nuts (saturated and trans fats are absolutely not allowed)

- Lean meat, like pork, skinless turkey, chicken breast and lean beef

- Fish such as snapper, halibut and salmon

- Shellfish, including clams, shrimp and mussels

- Meat from elk, bison, alligator and other nontraditional animal sources

- Fruits, limiting the amount of high sugar fruits like cherries, bananas and grapes if you are overweight

- Fruits such as avocados, plums, apples, berries, papaya and melon are allowed

- Fresh vegetables (in limited portions)

If you look at that list, you will see that modern man is going to have a tough time sticking to the caveman diet. Your body is unfortunately used to processed foods, dairy, unhealthy oils, sugar, salt and bad fat. Prehistoric man did not have those available, so you will not be eating them either.

The good news is, those items we just mentioned are the cornerstone of most human diseases. Since you will not be eating those foods, your risk of contracting cancer, gout, heart problems, diabetes, obesity and dangerously high cholesterol levels will start to drop almost immediately.

What Foods Are Not Allowed on the Caveman Diet?

From what we can tell, the caveman eat a fairly limited diet. Of course, none of today's manufacture red or processed foods were available then (and to the caveman's better health I might add).

If you abide strictly by the caveman, here is a list of "banned" items:

- Maltose

- Maple syrup

- Molasses

- Palm Sugar

- Raw sugar

- Rice Syrup

- Sorghum

- Sucrose

- Syrup

- Xylose

- Grains, including corn (sure, there were wild grains available to prehistoric man. But it actually made up an insignificant part of his diet.)

- Starchy foods like potatoes, beets, yams and cassava

- Peanuts, peas, beans and other legumes

- Dairy foods like cream, milk, yogurt, butter, cheese, ice cream, etc.

- Processed meats, such as bacon, sausage, deli meats and hot dogs

- Corn, cottonseed, peanut, soybean, rice bran and wheat germ oils (including foods like mayonnaise, which contains some of those oils)

- Salt

Our ancestral cave dwellers didn't have the chance to eat chili cheese fries with extra salt chased down with a large soda, and you cannot either!

But Doesn't a Plant-Based Diet Mean Eating Some of These Banned Foods?

Although all people on a plant-based diet should try to avoid processed and unnatural foods, the area of concern for vegetarians and vegans will be that grains, legumes and starches are not recommended.

Do not worry. This is where special adaptations come in (you'll find them later in this guide). Before we get to that, though, let's learn some more about the Paleo diet benefits.

Let's learn some more about the Paleo diet benefits.

The Benefits of a Paleo Diet

Limiting, and possibly totally eliminating, the chance of contracting cancer or some some kind of heart disease is a huge benefit of the prehistoric diet plan. If you only adopted this nutritional eating approach for those reasons, that is certainly good enough. But there are other benefits that you will enjoy as well, such as the following.

You Won't Develop an Unhealthy Processed Food Addiction

This is huge. You are probably well aware that many companies that market processed foods do not care if their products are killing you or not. They only want 2 things - 1) to make "food" as cheaply as possible, and 2) to make that so-called food as addictive as possible.

Sugar and salt are 2 of the most addictive and unhealthy chemicals found in processed foods. Unhealthy MSG is also very tasty, and unfortunately found in 60% to 75% of all processed foods. Tons of other 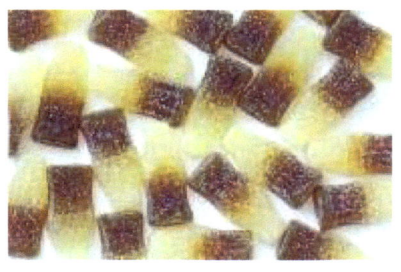 chemicals, sweeteners and unnatural additives make processed food cheap, incredibly tasty and addictive. This diet helps you avoid developing those dangerous addictions.

Your Muscle Mass Goes Up and Your Fat Content Goes Down

Who wouldn't be happy to burn fat and build muscle simply by changing what you eat? Seriously, you do not even have to change your level of physical fitness right now (although physical activity is highly encouraged as a healthy practice).

A high protein, low carbohydrate diet full of tasty, natural foods leads to muscle development by itself. The bigger and stronger your muscles are, the harder your metabolism has to work to fuel those muscles with energy. This naturally begins a fat burning and muscle building cycle that you are going to love.

You Only Eat "Good" Calories

If you want to be healthy and regulate your natural body weight, you need to eat a certain amount of calories each day. But when you ingest a lot of "empty" calories, you are definitely not healthy. Empty calories are those which deliver little to no nutritional value, like sugar and vegetable oil.

What liquid did your cave living ancestors drink 99% of the time? Pure water. He didn't slug down a 64-ounce soda, packed full of empty calories. All the calories you eat on the Paleo diet are filled with nutrition, not garbage.

You Will Have More Natural Energy

Empty calories, sugar, coffee and other energy boosting modern day foods and drinks inevitably leave you crashing. That short burst of energy is followed by a drained feeling and a lack of motivation or energy to do just about anything. The foods you eat when you follow the prehistoric diet plan are packed full of energy. They are natural foods, and your body naturally understands how to use them to regulate high energy levels throughout the day.

You Feel Full Longer

Nutrient dense foods deliver a minimal amount of calories in an extremely high level of nutritional goodness. Especially when compared to unhealthy oils and processed foods. So your body is happy after you eat, and it tells your brain so. According to some doctors and nutritionists, today's processed foods contain as little as 10% of the nutrients originally found in the food used to make that processed item.

This is why you get hunger cravings all day long, sometimes even just a short period after you are through eating some nutritionally poor modern day meal. That leads to overeating. This does not happen with the Paleolithic diet.

You Avoid Certain Diseases

The prehistoric diet is high on anti-inflammatory foods, wonderful antioxidants, phytonutrients and natural minerals. That means you dramatically reduce your risk of contracting the debilitating conditions we mentioned earlier, like high cholesterol, obesity, high blood pressure, heart disease and diabetes.

Is the Paleo Diet Safe for Everyone?

If you are pregnant, you may be rightfully concerned about whether the caveman diet is a healthy way to make it through this very important time in your life. You also may be wondering if children or elderly members of your family should attempt this nutritional approach.

Just think about this. You were here right now because he is. Humans enjoyed a very healthy diet the Paleolithic era. Remember, cancer, diabetes, heart problems and other diseases the natural inventions of modern man. They simply did not exist for prehistoric man.

So if you want to raise your children on this healthy diet, go ahead. The same is true if you are over 50, or pregnant, and was to incorporate the Paleo diet into your nutrition plans. However, you should always seek the advice of a physician and get a checkup before making any drastic dietary changes. This is true though matter what your age, or what type of physical condition you are is, and whether you are pregnant or not.

Paleo Diet Changes for Lacto-Ovo Vegetarians

If you are a lacto-ovo vegetarian, you eat a plant-based diet with no meat. In that sense, you are a vegetarian. But you also recognize eggs and dairy as a part of a healthy diet. Eggs and dairy are not a part of a strict caveman diet adherence. So as a lacto-ovo vegetarian, what diet changes can you adopt from the Paleo eating plan?

The "Protein Problem"

Well, the number one "problem" with any type of vegetarian diet plan is ensuring you get enough protein. One issue that some vegetarians find with the traditional Paleo diet is that their favorite protein sources – for example soya and tofu – are simply not 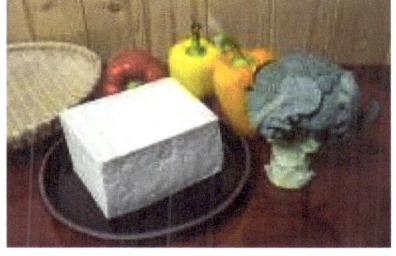 allowed. These were not consumed by our ancestors, and are considered processed foods (despite the health benefits). However, it's easy to get your protein elsewhere.

The truth is that as long as you eat sensibly, fruits, vegetables and grains can provide more than enough protein for the typical human. However, not all of these items are allowed on the Paleo diet.

The Vegetarian Solution

For vegetarians, one solution is quite easy. You can simply eat more eggs. Note, however, that the Paleo diet usually recommends eating them in moderation. Eggs, however, are an easy "Paleo" way to get more protein into your diet. However, they certainly do not match the amount of protein you'd get by eating meat.

Hummus

Of all the plant-based foods that can really knock up your protein, hummus is probably the most well-known. While it's primarily a dip made and eaten in Egypt, hummus has become a staple part of many diets in the western world, usually bought prepackaged. Along with tahini, olive oil, salt and lemon juice, cooked chickpeas are mashed into a puree that goes well with a flatbread or similar food. It's mainly had as a snack in the west, but can also be used as part of or as the whole main meal. Most of you will have had it by now, but if you haven't you really need to get it into your diet.

The usual ingredient in hummus is chickpeas, which is the real star of this food, is filled with high levels of fiber, B vitamins, manganese and obviously contains huge amounts of protein. If made yourself, hummus can be made with absolutely no salt or reduced amount of anything that is deemed negative such as the high fat tahini oil. While it's almost always low in calories, you have to be careful that any pre-packaged hummus that you buy for the plant-based protein isn't also filled with high levels of salt or even sugar.

Hummus is often eaten as a snack, but that doesn't mean there isn't numerous ways that the delicious food can be eaten.

We've thrown some ideas together to get you started on your way to a diet rich in hummus and low in meat.

Many people choose to use hummus instead of butter in sandwiches or various other snacks, something that is open to you. A perfect addition to a cheese toastie is both sides of the toast covered in hummus before you stick it in the pan. Perfection.

The main thing that hummus is eaten with is falafel. Whether you put them both in a wrap, eat them both on top of a salad or even just have hot falafel with hummus on the side, they got together brilliantly.

If you make your own hummus, there are ways to make it thicker by addition, something you can check online. With this, you can marinade things such as roast vegetables before putting them on the side with a flatbread and even more hummus to dip.

As you can see from this short list, there are many ways you can bring hummus into your diet. If you're interested, want to get started making your own and think hummus sounds like the perfect addition to meal where meat is starting to lack, give the internet a search where you'll find hundreds of meals that use hummus.

The Vegan Solution

Vegans strictly forbid the consumption of animal food products. Hardcore vegans will not own, purchase or wear any type of item which was made from some part of an animal or animal byproduct.

Obviously, the Paleo diet is big on scarfing down lean meats, fish and shellfish.

So what is a vegan to do if he or she wants to experiment with the Paleolithic approach to nutrition? The answer is to adapt certain parts of the Paleo diet.

Adapting the Paleo Diet for Vegans and Vegetarians

To get the correct ratio of healthy proteins to fats and carbs, there is no question that the Paleo diet will need to be adapted for those who prefer to consume plant-based ingredients only. And this is not necessarily a bad thing at all – keep reading to find out more below.

Option 1: Changing the Rules for Grains and Legumes

The most common approach to a plant-based Paleo diet is to change the rules when it comes to grains and legumes. Of course, die-hard Paleo diet followers will not call this a true Paleo diet, and that's fine. It's a **modified Paleo diet**, for those who do not believe in consuming animal products.

Lentils

Yet another legume that vegans rely on in many ways, lentils are a perfect way to get protein from a plant-based snack without having to resort to meat. This edible has been used for years, having been part of the human diet for centuries now, so your body should have no issue digesting them.

They vary in both size and color, offering the chance to create many different meals due to its versatile nature. Like all plant-based foods that are high in protein, lentils come with huge levels of nutrition that you wouldn't normally get from meat, so there's many reason to start throwing it into your diet.

Along with the impressive amounts of protein, lentils also include essential nutrients like dietary fiber and micronutrients including folate, thiamine, phosphorus, iron and zinc. Lentils are regularly used by those suffering with diabetes as they have low levels of digestible starch and high levels of slowly digested starch. All you need to do to become part of the group enjoying their lentil hit is cook them from anywhere between ten and forty minutes to create a variety of meals.

They can be used to make healthy curries such as dahl or create a soup, adding in vegetables where it seems natural to add a little color and taste to the earthy legume. Once again, these things were once considered the food of peasants, but this usually meant they were high in nutrition, inexpensive and very easy to prepare.

We've taken it upon ourselves to suggest a few meal ideas you might enjoy that use lentils so you can start to throw away that dangerous meat and turn to lentils for your protein, improving your diet in no time.

If you're looking for an easy way to get those lentils into your body in the form of an easy snack or a food you can take out into the world, then you can make a red lentil soup. Not only can you spice it up with some chili or keep it light and fragrant, add in some vegetables to up the health benefits.

Another light snack that is high on the nutrients and various other positive effects is a salad that includes lentils. In the place of meat, you can also add in falafel to give it an extra texture and beef it up a little bit.

Buying lentils with the shell still intact will keep them together rather than bleeding out into a lovely puree, which means you can flavor them how you want and roll them into balls or bake them into lines. With these you can make anything, including wraps and sandwiches with a side of hummus or vegetables.

Once you've got your head around the lentil, you can start to experiment yourself, or look online to find out how other people eat their lentils and get them into their diets.

Grains

Under the regular Paleo diet, grains are not allowed due to the fact that they can cause a number of digestive and health problems for many of us.

However, all grains are not created equal. There are a number of "grain-like seeds" that vegans and vegetarians will want to include in their modified Paleo diet. Traditionally these ingredients are still not allowed in the Paleo diet, because they tend to behave similarly to grains, and are mostly carbs.

However, nutritionists agree that ingredients like quinoa, amaranth and buckwheat are a healthy addition to the diet. They can be used in the place of rice, and you may even find pastas and flours made from these ingredients to keep your diet a bit more interesting.

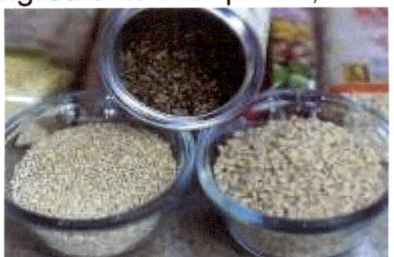

As long as you get enough protein in your diet, you can also start to include these healthy grain-like ingredients. The bonus is they will also help towards your protein intake.

Quinoa

Up until a few years ago, many people in the western world hadn't heard of quinoa, the crop only making its way across when people realized how it could be used in a diet as a highly nutritious plant-based protein. In particular, vegans and vegetarians latched onto it, as their diets can often struggle for protein when compared to the more traditional diet of those who eat meat and dairy. That being said, there's no need for quinoa to be enjoyed only by people who feel they must live off a strict diet, a valid plant-based protein for anyone looking to up their nutrition levels while also keeping their diet as healthy as possible.

For those who don't know what quinoa is, it is a pseudo cereal in that it isn't a grass, which all true cereals are. While you can also eat the leaves that grow off their plant, they're not widely commercially available, so it's the seeds that people tend to put into their diet to get some plant-based protein that they're missing out somewhere else. Not only are they high in protein, they also contain large amounts of essential amino acids that include lysine.

As we said earlier, this food is seen as a high end which can be seen hugely in these levels of nutritional value.

When it comes to figuring out how to get the stuff into your diet, then you'll have to start looking for some interesting little meals to reap the health benefits. We've compiled some of them below.

You can throw quinoa into a smoothie, meaning it's easy to get it down you in a snack and drink it throughout the day, not just at home.

If you're eating salads regularly, which you should be, you also add quinoa to these which should add a little texture to the meal while also filling you up with more nutrients than was already contained within the veg.

Quinoa can be used in the place of rice, boiling quite easily to be used either for stuffing vegetables or alongside a curry as you would pilau rice. You can also add in some vegetables or spices as long as you make sure it's not adding many calories.

For those regularly eating veggie or meat wraps, mixing in some quinoa will yet again add quite a good bit of texture while also increasing the taste burst you get from every bite.

As you can see, there's quite a lot that you can do to try and get quinoa into your diet, and that's just a few of the options open to you. If you take a look throughout the internet, you'll find that there's numerous recipes open to you. Once you're enjoying quinoa to the point where you don't have to sneak it into your own food, you can start to get experimental, creating your own healthy meals to make sure that you don't get bored of this superfood.

Along with a other plant-based proteins, you'll find that there's enough to be creating enough large meals to keep you going for a while.

Hopefully you can see from this article that quinoa is a very welcome addition to any diet, that the grain is not only suitable for those struggling to go protein into a restricted diet but also for anyone looking for a high protein food that is plant-based.

While it may have a certain reputation, gathered after the western world took the food over as a middle class health food rather than the peasant food filled with nutrition that it once was, there's nothing wrong with some quinoa indulgence. These little seeds are worth a second look, so don't judge them on what others say before you've given them a chance yourself with one of our suggested meals. You won't be let down.

Amaranth

Many of life's perfections are created and found in nature. Beautiful gems, medicines and perhaps most importantly, food and water, are found in nature ready and waiting for us to come and harvest them. Amaranth is one such food cultivated by nature to be highly nutritious, versatile, and chocked full of health benefits for both physical and mental wellbeing.

Such foods cannot be manmade or otherwise synthetically produced, which makes these nature made wonder foods something you should be adding to your diet immediately.

What Is Amaranth?

Amaranth, or amaranthus, refers to over 60 species of tall, green plants that sport vibrant purple, red, or gold flowers. Its name comes from the Greek 'amarantos' which means 'unfading' or 'one that does not fade.'

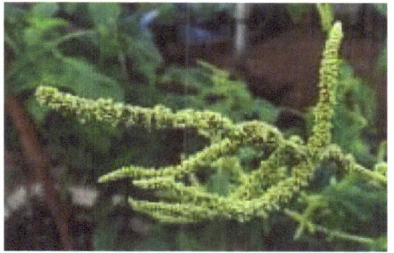

This plant certainly lives up to its name for the flowers are as vibrant and beautiful as ever, even after they have been harvested and dried. Often found as a beautiful member of showy gardens, amaranth has been around for centuries. It was a staple for the Aztec Empire and was used for both food and ceremonial reasons.

While it is commonly thought of as a cereal grain, amaranth is not exactly a "true" whole grain. However thanks to its glowing nutrient profile, it is often lumped together with other cereals due to its versatility.

Health Benefits of Amaranth

It's Chocked Full of Vitamins and Minerals: There is a long and winding list of health benefits found in amaranth that do wonders for the body. Amaranth contains over three times the average amount of calcium than most plant foods and is also a great source of potassium, phosphorous, iron and magnesium. These nutrients are important for regulating your appetite, building strong bones, cleansing, and oxygenating the blood, and a host of other housekeeping functions for bodily systems.

This is also the only grain that has been shown to contain vitamin C, which is well known for boosting the immune system and aiding in the fight against disease and illnesses.

It's An Excellent Source of Protein: Amaranth is also an excellent source of protein. It contains much more protein than most other grains and contains lysine, which is an amino acid often missing from whole grains. When added to a diet, amaranth offers boosted energy levels and promotes bowel regularity and a healthy metabolism. It also contains lunasin, a peptide that was previously identified in soybeans and was thought to help prevent cancer as well as reduce inflammation that is present with certain chronic health conditions such as heart disease, stroke, and diabetes.

It Promotes Heart Health: Studies have shown that amaranth is a whole grain that can potentially lower cholesterol effectively. Through various studies conducted over the last decade, findings have shown that, when fed to chickens, the amount of bad cholesterol in the body was lowered significantly. This study was duplicated in Canada, the U.S., and Russia, and each study offered similar results. While promising, whether or not amaranth will have the same effect on human's remains to be seen. However, it can't hurt to add this to your daily heart-healthy regimen.

It's Gluten-Free: Today, gluten-free diets are extremely popular and widely sought after. Those with Celiac disease must follow them, but those without Celiac disease have also found them to be a healthy option in their lives. Many find that cutting out gluten makes them feel better, lighter, and more alert.

Luckily, adding amaranth to your gluten-free diet is easy and it can be used as a great substitute for other grains used in dough to increase elasticity and allow for leavening.

Make This Extremely Versatile Plant A Part Of Your Lifestyle

For centuries, amaranth has been used by humans for a number of different reasons. In addition to the listed health benefits, just about every inch of this plant can be used for something.

The seed is an excellent source of protein and is easy to cook and the seed flour is ideal for healthy baked goods. The leaves, roots, and stems are also consumed as leafy veggies in many parts of the world and used for cooking and various dishes. They can be steamed, mashed, or simply seasoned and added to a favorite dish.

In addition to being used as food, the amaranth plant is also used for aesthetic reasons. The gorgeous flowers of this plant have been widely used for dyes—specifically as a source of a deep red dye that comes from the flowers. It is also used for ornamental reasons in gardens or in homes and is grown for both its beauty and its many uses.

Buckwheat

Time and again nature reminds us just how good it is at creating nutritious and healthful food for humans to consume. Why so many of us reach for factory made junk is a mystery, when we have at our disposable nature's perfect plant food gems, and buckwheat is a perfect example.

What is Buckwheat?

Agriculturists refer to it as a pseudo cereal. While the name leads one to believe the buckwheat plant yields a grain, the fruit of a grass plant with a hard exterior or hull, it does not.

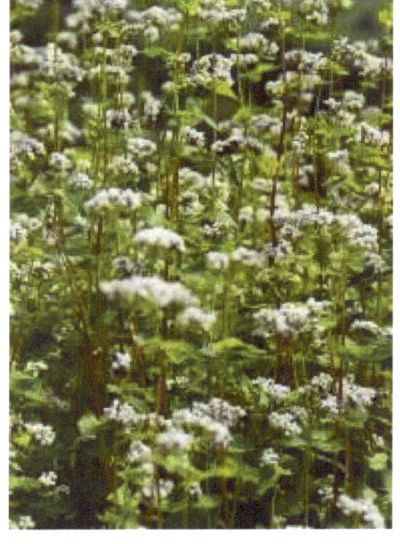

It is actually a type of shrub-like plant native to the temperate regions of East Asia. The buckwheat plant is bright green, having broad heart-shape leaves and white flowers, and its seeds are harvested for use.

The plant tends to be short and broad, easily forming a notable level of ground coverage. Its cultivation in China dates back to 1,000 AD.

Currently, buckwheat is cultivated worldwide with most of it growing in China, Japan, and North America. Over 14 species of the plant exist with two of them being cultivated species and the remaining existing in the wild.

Nutritional Content

Buckwheat contains a rich nutritional profile of protein, minerals, and fiber.

The levels of copper, zinc, and manganese exceed the levels found in other cereal grains. The significant bioavailability of copper, zinc, and potassium also makes buckwheat a desirable addition to any diet. In addition, buckwheat does not contain gluten so people with gluten sensitivities or intolerance may safely consume pure buckwheat flour, groats, and grits.

The protein content of buckwheat exceeds that of oats, one of the best plant sources for protein. Its protein content includes all eight essential amino acids with a strong concentration of lysine at six percent of its nutritional profile.

Buckwheat grains contain high quantities B-complex vitamins, especially riboflavin (vitamin B2) and niacin (vitamin B3).

The grains contain high levels of soluble and insoluble fiber, which helps with digestion and elimination.

Gluten free so ideal for those with Celiac Disease or gluten sensitivity.

Health Benefits

People derive many health benefits from adding buckwheat to their diet.

It is good for diabetics. The high fiber content slows the absorption of glucose in the bloodstream, helping to maintain healthy blood sugar levels and possibly lowering A1C.

It supports the immune system. Copper, zinc and potassium are key minerals for establishing and maintaining a healthy immune system. Copper also supports the production of red blood cells.

It helps heart health. The magnesium content of buckwheat assists with lowering blood pressure building balanced cholesterol levels.

Buckwheat fights inflammation a precursor and symptom of many systemic diseases. The polyphenols, water-soluble plant pigments with antioxidant properties, found in buckwheat combat inflammation and dysfunctional clotting in blood vessels.

Purchasing And Preparing

The seeds of the plant are harvested and processed in a variety of ways to make them available for various uses. After removing the hull from the three-sided triangular shaped seeds, they may be added to cereals, coarsely ground into grits, finely ground into flour or roasted to make kasha.

Preparation methods for buckwheat groats and kasha include boiling, steaming and baking. The dishes serve the same role in meals as potatoes or rice. Buckwheat flour may also be added to sauces and gravies to give thicken them and give them additional color.

Other uses for buckwheat include:

- Providing honey bees with nectar which they transform into a dark strongly flavored honey

- A component of livestock feed to be used in combination with corn, barley or oats

- As a cover crop to prevent weeds before planting another crop

- As a fertilizer crop to be plowed under to return nutrients and moisture to the soil prior to the next planting

Buckwheat is a versatile and nutritious plant. This gluten free and nutrient dense food grows quickly making it a plentiful food source. Some people get a skin rash when they eat buckwheat so monitor yourself for sensitivity.

Buckwheat is widely available and lends itself to a variety of preparations such as breakfast cereal, porridge pancakes as well as grain salads, pilafs, Asian Soba noodles, snacks and in baked goods.

If you find the flavor of buckwheat too heavy or bitter, try blending it with other grains.

Beans and Legumes

Some people claim that beans contain "lectins" or "phytates" that can create inflammation or impair mineral absorption, which is the reason why they are generally not recommended on the standard Paleo diet.

They key here is simply not to overdo things. Try limiting your bean consumption to around a cup per day, and monitoring how your body reacts (some people are more prone to digestive reactions than others).

Another great option is to eat soaked or sprouted legumes.
These are becoming easier and
easier to buy in stores, and you
can also do the soaking
yourself. This will help to
reduce the "anti-nutrient"
content. Going a step further,
you can sprout your legumes,
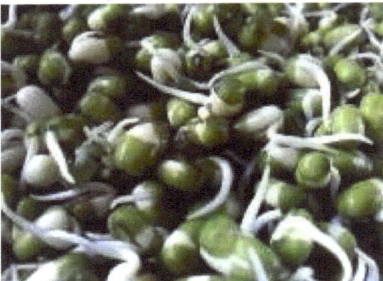
beans and seeds and eat the sprouts themselves.

Option 2: A Raw Vegan Diet

There are a group of vegans who are pretty much already
following a Paleo diet, simply without the meat. This is
known as a raw vegan diet, which combines the principles of
a raw diet with the vegan lifestyle of avoiding all animal
products and byproducts.

A raw vegan diet will be mostly based on eating large
quantities of raw vegetables and fruits, plus healthy fats and
nuts and seeds. Some eat sprouted or soaked grains and
legumes, whereas others cut this out entirely.

Option 3: Consuming a *Mostly* Plant-Based Diet

Although many vegetarians and vegans will not be open to
this idea, some people choose to combine a *mostly*-vegan
diet with a *mostly*-Paleo diet.

Dr. Mark Hyman is a doctor and bestselling author. He writes
frequently about how what you eat determines how you look
and feel, how healthy you are and how long you live. He
credits himself with making up the word **"pegan"** as a way to
explain his belief that a combination of Paleo and vegan
diets provides the best possible nutritional approach to smart
health.

All meat is not created equal. Grass-fed lean beef like lamb, poultry, venison and bison that is sustainably raised can be enjoyed in sensible portions as a part of a healthy diet. In fact, eating "clean" meat 2 or 3 times a week has been linked to healthy cholesterol levels, reduced belly fat and increased muscle mass.

Wild caught salmon, sardines, and mackerel deliver rich Omega 3 fats and DHA. You can get those wonderful natural components from algae, but it is in extremely high quantities in those fish we just mentioned. Healthy alpha linolenic acid (ALA) is found in plants, but you have to turn to some other source for Omega 3 fatty acids.

Pegan practitioners have found the following benefits by combining the best that Paleo and vegan approaches have to offer:

- Lower chances of contracting heart disease, cancer, diabetes, obesity and other deadly diseases

- Lower body fat and more muscle mass

- "All day" energy

- Healthy, young looking hair and skin

- Boosted mental process, clearer thinking and a reduced risk of contracting Alzheimer's and other neurological diseases

- Less stress and anxiety

The good news is that you can also experience the benefits of a Pegan diet by following a healthy fully-vegan diet, so don't feel as though you necessarily *need* to consume any of these animal products.

Are We Really Meant to Eat Meat?

The Paleo diet relies on the idea that humans were meant to eat meat. It's what our ancestors did, and it's what we should do to improve our health. In fact, everything about the Paleo diet is what our ancestors did.

However, this is just one school of thought. If you're reading this book, then you're probably open to the idea that humans were not necessarily made to eat meat. We all know that it is natural for humans to eat meat, but many scientific studies show that it is also natural and healthy for us to thrive on a plant-based diet.

Meat Associated Health Issues

To most people, protein is something you get from meat and nowhere else, a myth that keeps people away from vegan and vegetarian diets for fear of losing out on the optimal amount of protein. If you didn't already realize, there are many plant-based proteins that will allow you the nutrition levels you need while also staying healthy, meaning you've got nothing to worry about. Read on to see exactly what issues can be brought on by meat and why you should be moving to a far more plant-based diet.

Cancer

It's been long been believed that meat, processed red meat in particular, can increase the risk of cancer in anyone, with the World Health Organization confirming that they believe the same thing earlier this year.

With it confirmed by such a body, it's hard to ignore what was, until now, mainly just speculation made by tabloid newspapers based on improperly handled statistics. Now, it's held by most people that meat will be increasing your chances of many types of cancer, especially intestinal and prostate, every day that you continue to eat meat.

Heart Disease

Now this one has been known for years now, with many older men dying due to their high level of meat intake during their younger years. This is entirely avoidable, and it still baffles many as to why people still continue to eat their body weight in meat and wonder why then die of heart disease in their later life. The cholesterol in the meat, and also in many dairy products, will only help block your arteries and lead to eventual heart attack or stroke.

Erectile Dysfunction

We're afraid this one comes with less evidence than the others listed here, but it's still something that could make a lot of men turn from meat very quickly. Like cigarettes, the increase in cholesterol makes it harder for your blood to get to the extremities, which means that it'd make sense that you would suffer with erectile dysfunction with a diet filled with meat. Not only this but there's some evidence that a diet high in meat won't help men with their erectile issues due to their tendency to keep hormone levels unbalanced within the human body.

Issues With Weight

Studies have shown that people who have a diet that contains meat struggle to maintain a healthy body weight. While we believe that human beings have a right to decide what is a healthy weight for themselves, it has to be accepted that extreme weight can bring with it many health concerns, on both sides of the scale. Pulling meat out of your diet could not only help you lose weight in the short term, but it will also help you maintain that weight loss in the long term, something that we think is definitely worth it.

Higher Rate Of Illness

While it's a lie to say someone who lives a vegan or vegetarian diet can't also get ill from what they've eaten, meat is more likely to contain foodborne illnesses. These can make you severely ill and are definitely not something to be scoffed at. Once again, anyone can get ill from the food they consumes, but it's much more like to happen to those eating meat.

From the World Health Organization saying that red meat will cause cancer and the saturated fats leading to struggles concerning heart disease or weight gain, there's always reason to leave meat out of your diet. There really is an alternative to that meat you have in your diet, and often a plant-based protein or a filling grain can be the difference you need to get your eating patterns in balance while throwing away anything that is dangerous to your body working properly.

If you're worried about the negative effects that eating meat can have on your body, then don't worry because there's always an alternative.

The meat that we eat now is far from natural and the way it would have been when our ancestors ate it. The meats back then would have come from wild animals, not from factory farmed animals that are fed a completely unnatural diet and are given unnatural antibiotics. Grass-fed meats 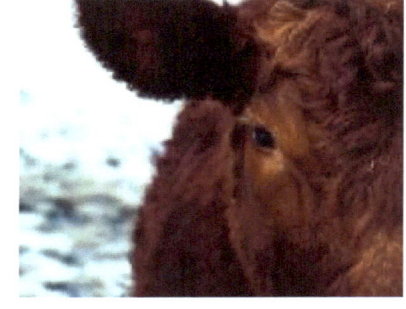 may be considered more natural, but they are still far removed from what our ancestors ate.

Further to that, many vegetarians and vegans do not mind going against what used to be natural. Often this is a lifestyle choice, and not one that solely revolves around diet.

If you have seen the documentary "Cowspiracy" then you will know how much of an impact animal agriculture has on our fragile environment (even so-called "sustainable" grass-fed beef). And many of us just no longer want to be a part of animal suffering.

The truth is that even those who adhere strictly to the original Paleo diet will never truly eat like a caveman. So much has changed that it is truly impossible. The way we get our meat and vegetables has changed, and our genes have changed.

As Professor Marlene Zuk, an evolutionary biologist at the University of Minnesota, puts it:

"The Paleo diet is based on the idea that human genetics have not changed or evolved over the past 10,000 years, since the time before the use of agriculture, but plenty of evidence exists that our genes have changed over the last few thousand years, and these changes mean we can eat foods our hunter-gatherer ancestors could not."

Conclusion

Prehistoric man ate a lot of nuts and berries. He also ate copious amounts of meat, fruit and leafy greens. He benefited from the healthy fats found in avocados, fish like salmon, olives and coconuts. He was almost never overweight, and was certainly not obese. Human life was not hampered by debilitating and deadly conditions like cancer, heart disease, obesity and diabetes.

Men and women in the Paleolithic era began bonding together in groups, and created the first human societies. They lived and ate naturally, and that is what the Paleo diet is all about.

Can you incorporate the Paleolithic diet into your vegan or vegetarian beliefs?

Sure, why not. Vegans, vegetarians and caveman diet practitioners all agree on one thing ... today's processed, salted, fast food, sugar-filled approach to nutrition is deadly.

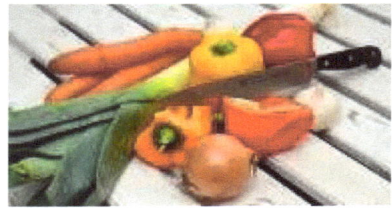

So add Paleo diet practices to your vegetarian lifestyle, however strictly you feel is best for you and for the environment and/or the animals. The Paleo police are not going to show up at your door and chastise you because you changed a rule here or there.

And don't forget to take it easy on yourself. Enjoying a non-Paleo food item once or twice a week is probably not going to kill you.

Just don't "reward" yourself with unhealthy processed foods on a regular basis. You may even find that, once your body gets used to eating a prehistoric diet, your cravings for chocolate, cheese and sugar will disappear.

Plant-Based Paleo Ingredients — Checklist

Print this checklist so you can easily refer to it when getting used to your new diet!

PALEO FOODS THAT ARE ALREADY PLANT-BASED:

☐ Eggs (if you are vegetarian - no more than 6 to 12 per week)

☐ Nuts and seeds (under 4 ounces a day if trying to lose weight)

☐ Healthy fats, e.g. olive oil, coconut oil, avocados and nuts

☐ Fruits such as avocados, plums, apples, berries, papaya and melon

☐ If overweight, limited high sugar fruits e.g. cherries, bananas, grapes

☐ Fresh vegetables

FOODS THAT AREN'T NORMALLY PALEO, BUT GOOD FOR VEGANS:

☐ Grain-like seeds such as quinoa, amaranth and buckwheat

☐ Soaked and sprouted beans and legumes

IF YOU WISH TO OCCASIONALLY INCLUDE ANIMAL PRODUCTS:

☐ Lean meat, e.g. pork, skinless turkey, chicken breast and lean beef

☐ Fish such as snapper, halibut and salmon

☐ Shellfish, including clams, shrimp and mussels

☐ Meat from elk, bison, alligator and other nontraditional animal sources

PLANT-BASED/ VEGETARIAN FOODS TO AVOID AT ALL TIMES:

☐ Refined sugar, plus honey, molasses, maple syrup etc.

☐ Grains, including corn, wheat and rice

☐ Dairy foods like cream, milk, yogurt, butter, cheese, ice cream, etc.

☐ Processed plant-based meats

☐ Corn, cottonseed, peanut, soybean, rice bran and wheat germ oils

☐ Salt

Other Senior Health and Fitness Books by This Author

If you would like to read more about Senior Health and Fitness, here is a list of the titles, CreateSpace links and descriptions:

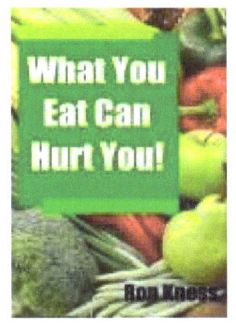

What You Eat Can Hurt You

https://www.createspace.com/4963196

Do you know that certain foods increase your risk for inflammation, disease and illness? It's true! And certain foods can help cure and heal you if you do get sick. Knowing which foods to eat and which ones to avoid empowers you to manage your own health.

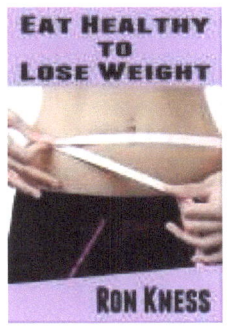

Eat Healthy to Lose Weight

https://www.createspace.com/4962939

As you read through our book, we show you which foods you should and should not be eating to reach your weight loss goal, along with discussing how to maintain your weight loss and stay within a few pounds of your goal weight. Banish the weight you keep gaining back each time by learning how to live a healthy lifestyle.

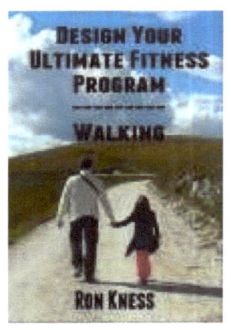

Design Your Ultimate Fitness Program - Walking

https://www.createspace.com/5252272

In my book Design Your Ultimate Fitness Program – Walking, we discuss the considerations that need to be made when designing a custom walking program, along with:
• Equipment needed
• Wearable technology you can use to track your walking
• And how to make walking more challenging

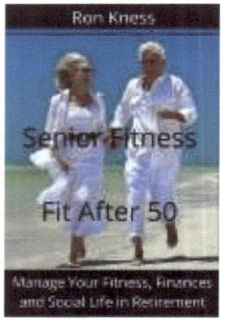

Senior Fitness – Fit After 50: Learn How to Manage Your Fitness, Finances and Social Life in Retirement

https://www.createspace.com/5474751

Inside you will discover answers to your most pressing questions:
• What do I need to know about downsizing my home?
• What are the best tips for staying healthy as you approach your 50's?
• When should I start planning for retirement?
• I am worried about being lonely once I retire, do others feel the same?
• Is it worthwhile to carry two homes during retirement?
And more…

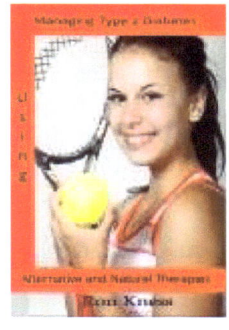

Managing Type 2 Diabetes Using Alternative And Natural Therapies

https://www.createspace.com/5401244

While Type 2 diabetes can be managed medically, there are many alternative natural and holistic methods of therapy and treatment that can further enhance quality of life and minimize the effects of this disease. In this book, I discuss 12 different types, including yoga, reflexology and acupuncture to name just three.

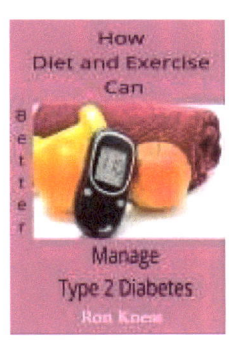

How Diet and Exercise Can Better Manage Type 2 Diabetes

https://www.createspace.com/5404845

Of the different types of diabetes, only Type 2 can be reversed. In my book How Diet and Exercise Can Better Manage Type 2 Diabetes, we reveal the three things you can do to best manage your disease, including:
• Diet
• Exercise
• Weight management

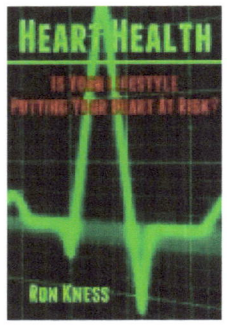

[Heart Health: Is Your Lifestyle Putting Your Heart at Risk?](#)

https://www.createspace.com/5464020

In my ebook Is Your Lifestyle Putting Your Heart At Risk? we discuss the six greatest risks to your heart and the lifestyle changes you can make to mitigate them.

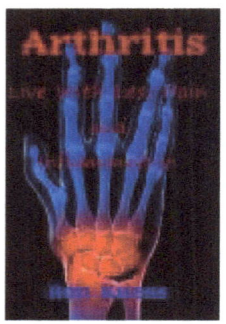

[Arthritis – Live Wth Less Pain and Inflammation: Tips and Techniques You Can Use to Lessen the Pain and Inflammation](#)

https://www.createspace.com/5457441

Discover Simple Tips & Information That Will Help Reduce The Painful Symptoms Of Arthritis!

You learn things like:
• Simple and effective information that will help you manage the pain and inflammation that comes along with arthritis, so that you can live an active, full life without debilitating pain.
• The different types of arthritis, their symptoms and how to alleviate their painful side effects.
• The pros and cons of over-the-counter arthritis medications, plus simple tips that will help you know how to choose the right supplements.

• Free, yet effective ways to get relief from arthritis pain and inflammation, so you don't have to suffer anymore.
the effects arthritis can have significant impact on your physical and mental well-being, but this books shows you how to overcome its painful symptoms and live life relatively pain free.

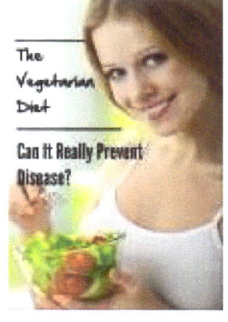

The Vegetarian Diet – Can It Really Prevent Disease?

https://www.createspace.com/5519874

Is a vegetarian diet right for you? Multiple studies have shown over and over that a vegetarian diet goes along way in preventing certain chronic diseases, such as:

• Heart Disease
• Cancer
• Diverticulitis
• Type 2 Diabetes
• Hypertension
• Obesity
• Kidney Failure

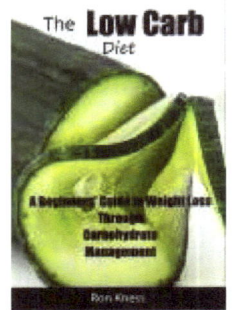

The Low Carb Diet: A Beginner's Guide to Weight Loss Through Carbohydrate Management

https://www.createspace.com/5416348

In my book "The Low-Carb Diet – A Beginners' Guide to Weight Loss Through Carbohydrate Management", I reveal a successful method of losing weight based in part on the amount and type of carbohydrates you consume.

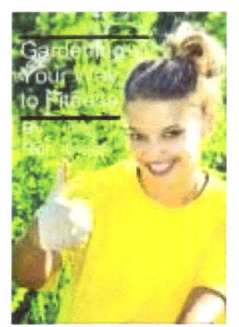

Gardening Your Way to Fitness: The Fun Way to Get Fit and Provide Beauty and Healthful Bounty for Your Family

https://www.createspace.com/5459564

The gym is a great place to stay fit during the colder seasons, but once the temperature turns warmer you want to spend more time outside. Plus, you'll have the benefit of fresh wholesome produce to enjoy by growing vegetables in your backyard garden.

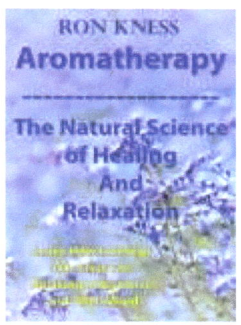

Aromatherapy - The Science of Healing and Relaxation: Learn How Essential Oils Elicit The Relaxation Response And Alter Mood

https://www.createspace.com/5714434

In my book Aromatherapy – The Science of Healing and Relaxation, we reveal the natural holistics methods you can use to heal the body from certain medical issues and to relive stress through relaxation. In particular we talk about:
• Aromatherapy - what it is and how it works
• Essential Oils – how the effects of certain aromas differs from others
• Recipes – how to make your own essential oil combinations

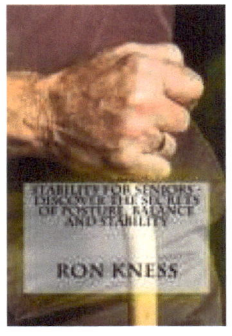

Stability for Seniors: Discover the Secrets of Posture, Balance and Stability

https://www.createspace.com/6096479

Many people sacrifice their health in pursuit of their career. They are so busy making a living that they neglect to make a life. The excuse that they do not have time to exercise is tossed about so frequently that they end up letting their health and fitness slide.

If you are not regularly active, you will have muscular atrophy over time. Your flexibility will decrease. Your core strength will diminish. As time progresses, you will be less limber and more rigid.

This is exactly how people age poorly. It's a process that has snowballed over time.

Only with regular exercise and a healthy diet can you have a body that is fit and has the ability to almost reverse aging.

If you have neglected your health for years and life seems to be a chore now because you can't get around without assistance, do not feel dejected.

You can remedy the situation. You can restore the strength, balance and stamina that you have lost. It is never too late to become what you might have been.

This guide will show you exactly what you need to do to restore your balance, strengthen your core and give you the ability to live life to its fullest. Read how …

About the Author

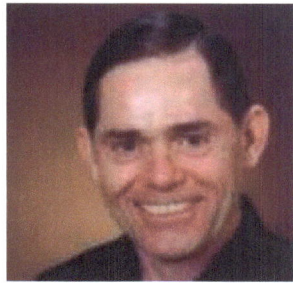 I grew up in Central Minnesota, where my parents owned and operated a fishing resort. Once out of high school I tried a couple of semesters of college, only to quit halfway through the Spring term; I decided at that time that college wasn't for me.

Then I decided to follow my father's previous occupation as an auto mechanic. I graduated from a two-year of vocational training course and worked as a mechanic. While in vocational training, I decided to join the National Guard where I eventually ended up working full-time for 32 years.

So how does all of this relate to writing? In one of my leadership schools, the instructor, who was an English teacher at a juvenile detention center, presented writing to me in a whole new way - a way that started to develop my interest in working with words.

Fast forward about 40 years and I now have over 50 books listed on Amazon for Kindle and CreateSpace.

Besides my own writing, I also ghostwrite ebooks, reports, articles, blogs and do Kindle conversions for my clients on a variety of topics.

Today my wife and I live in Gold Canyon, AZ, where you'll find me happily sitting in my office typing away on my laptop as I work on my next book or ghostwriting project . . . that is if we are not traveling on a cruise ship - our new-found mode of travel.

www.ingramcontent.com/pod-product-compliance
Lightning Source LLC
Chambersburg PA
CBHW040314010626
45792CB00022B/303